SHERMAN'S SHAKES

Written by
Garrett & Amy Sacco

Illustrated by
Garrett Sacco

I know them!

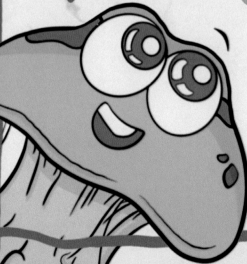

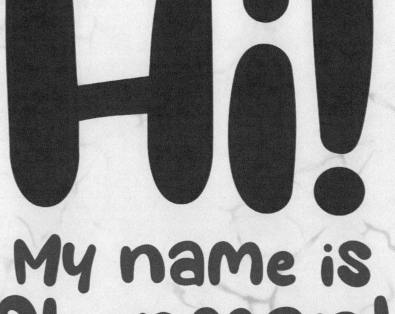

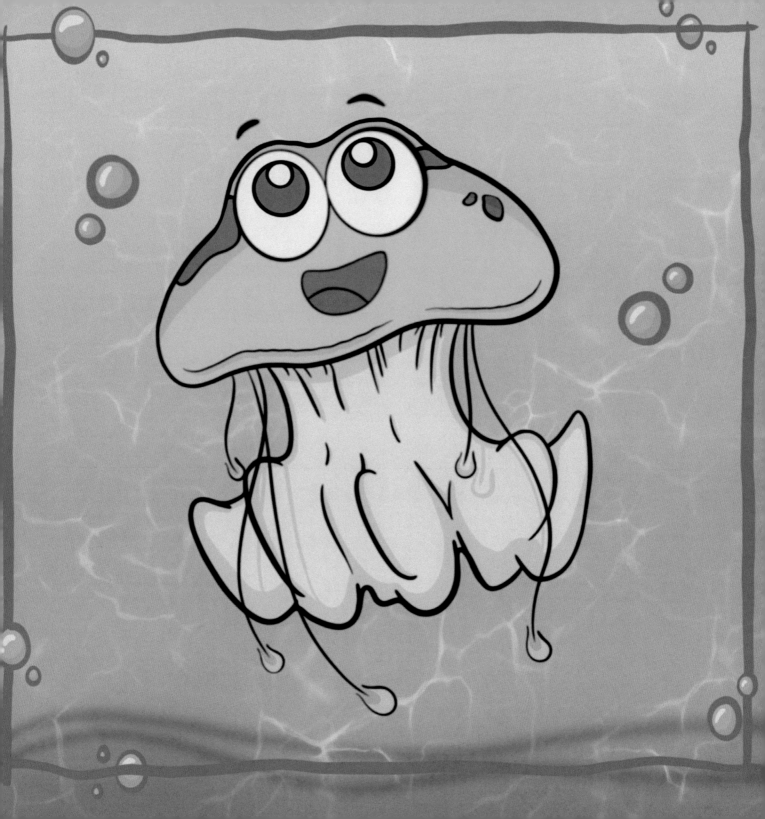

I go to school in
the big open sea
I love my family
and friends,
and they love me

I have a little story
that I'd like to tell,
My hope is that it
can help you as well

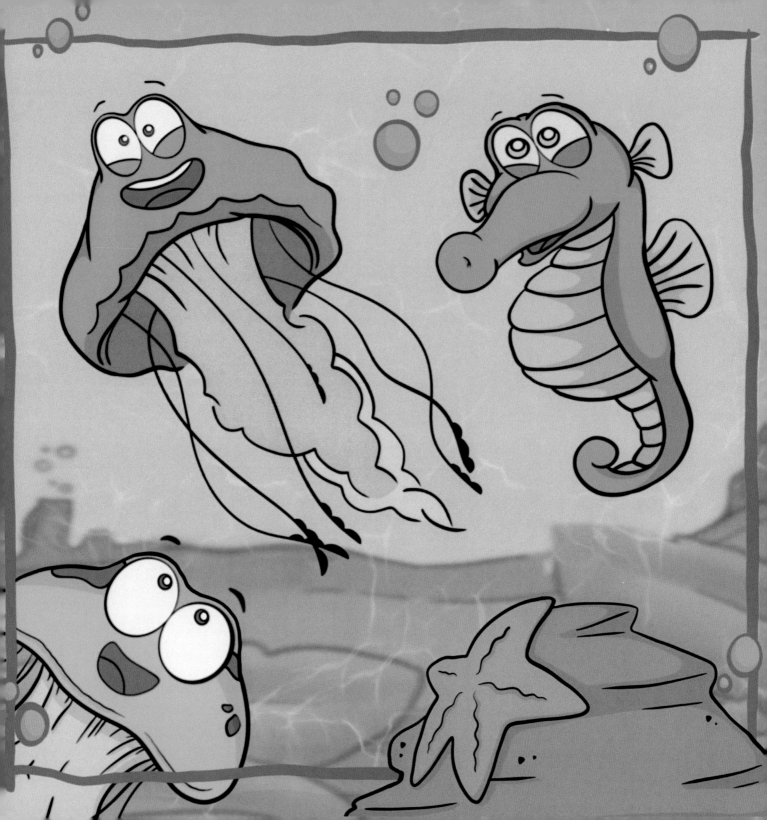

One day at school,
all warm and sunny,

I had a sudden
feeling, and it felt
kind of funny

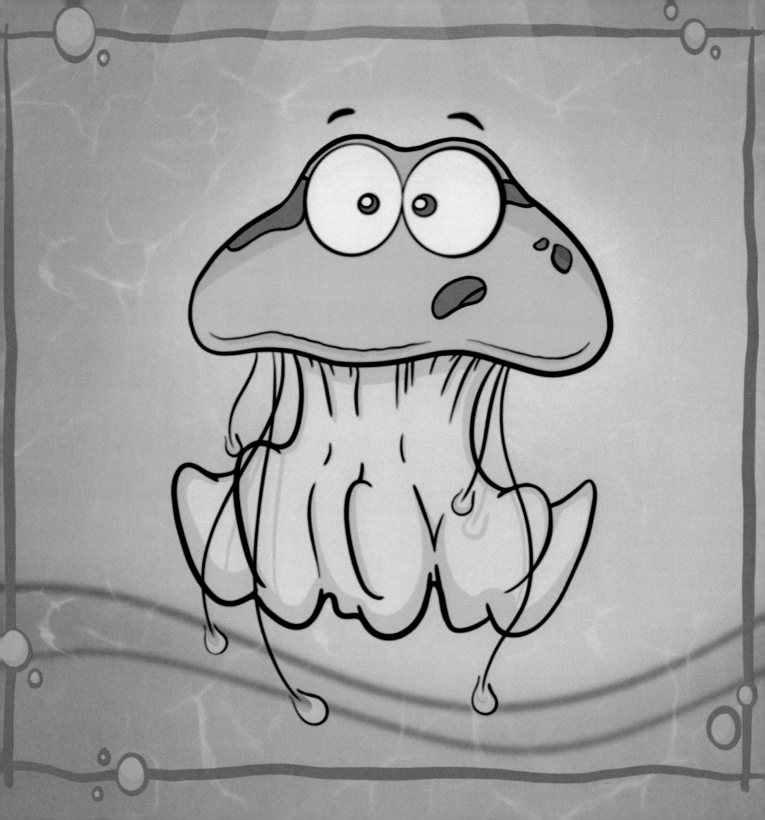

My tummy and head
felt woozy and sore,
like a big ocean wave
swelling up on the shore

I was a little confused
and a little bit scared
I think this has happened
before, but I was
not prepared

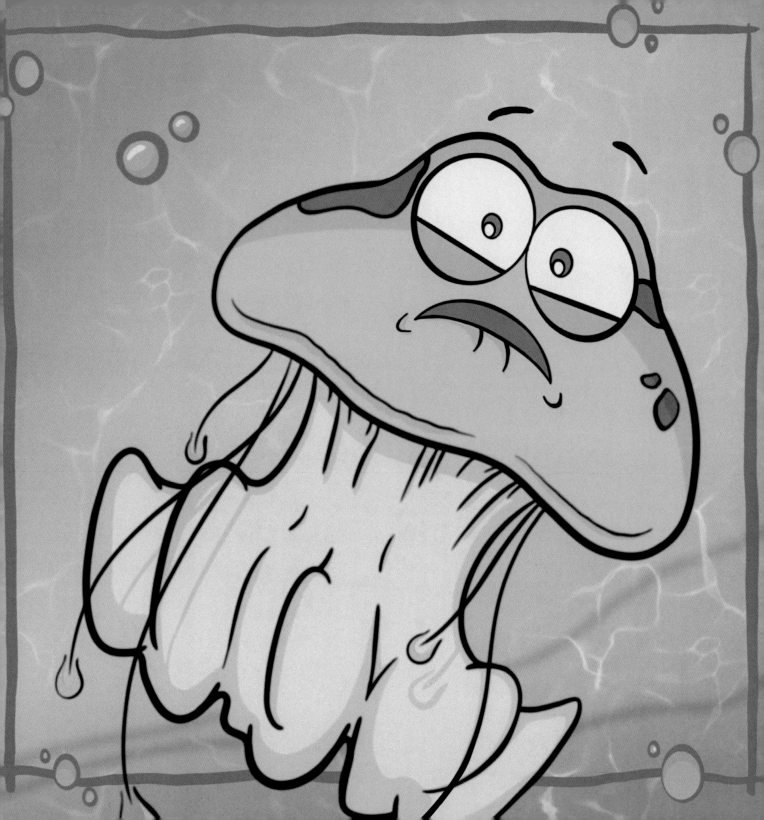

Then all of a sudden, without much of a break,

I started to tingle... I started to SHAKE!

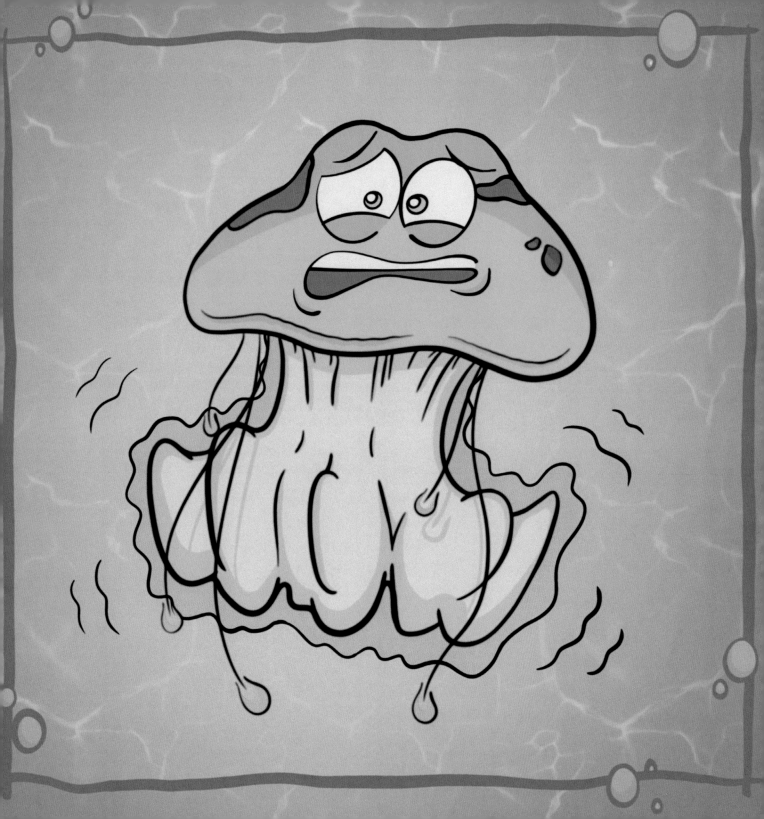

What happened
next, I don't
know at all,

But my teacher
Ms. Shelly helped
me stay calm

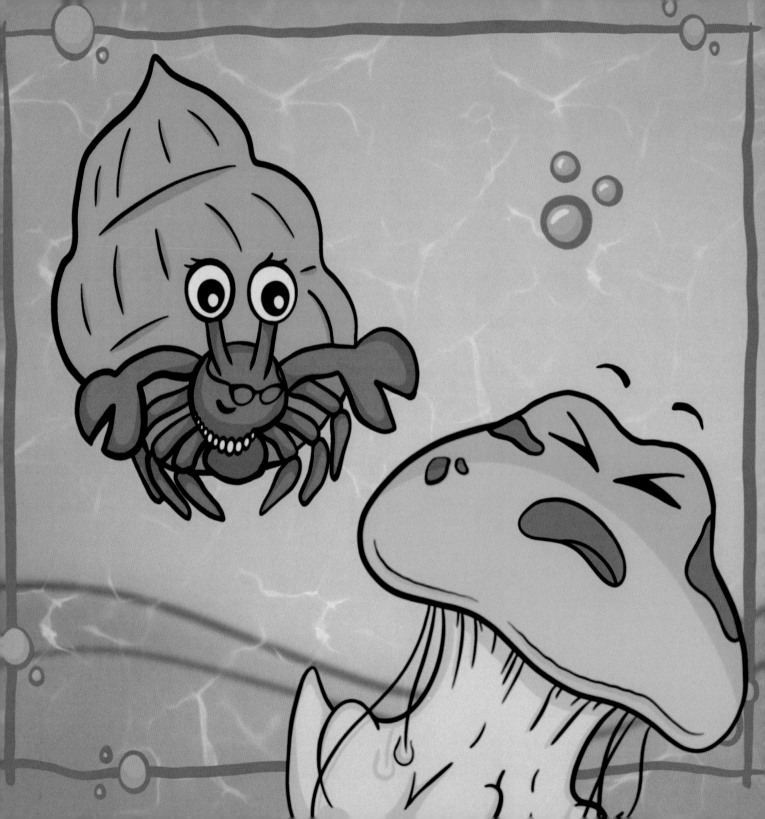

Today, I went to
the doctor;
Doctor Octopus
is his name!

"I am a neurologist"
he said, "a doctor
for the brain!"

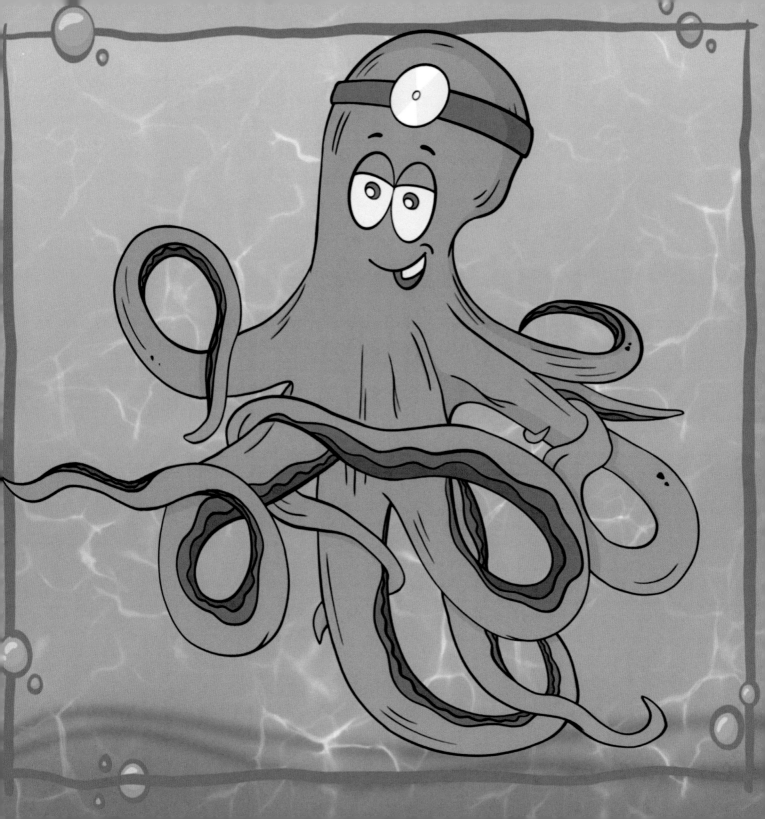

"In all of our brains,"
said Doc, "there is
great power, like
lightning in the sky,
or rain in a shower!"

"Most special of all,"
he said with a wink,
"there is ELECTRICITY
to help us see, feel,
speak, move, & think!"

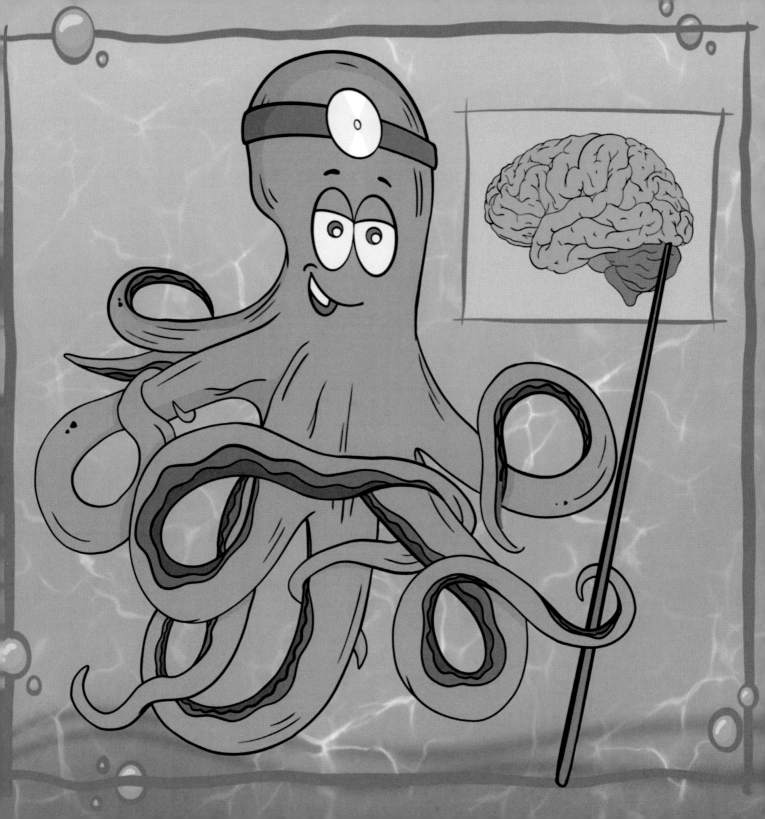

Our brains can do many things, and they can do them very quick

Doc told me that my brain is EXTRA ELECTRIC!

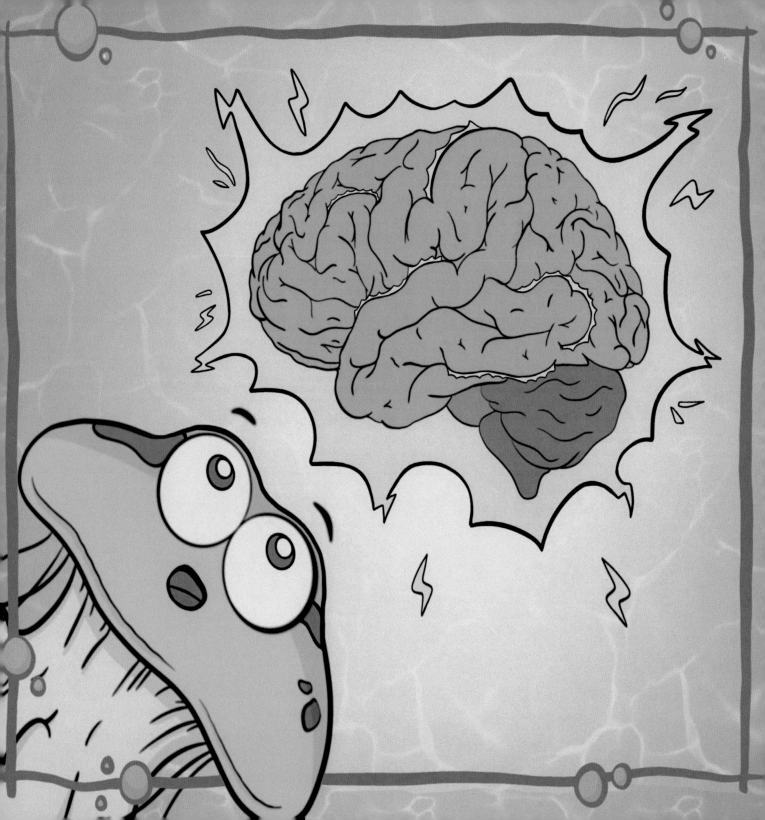

There is sometimes extra electricity that my brain makes

This means sometimes I might have SEIZURES... the doctor word for the SHAKES!

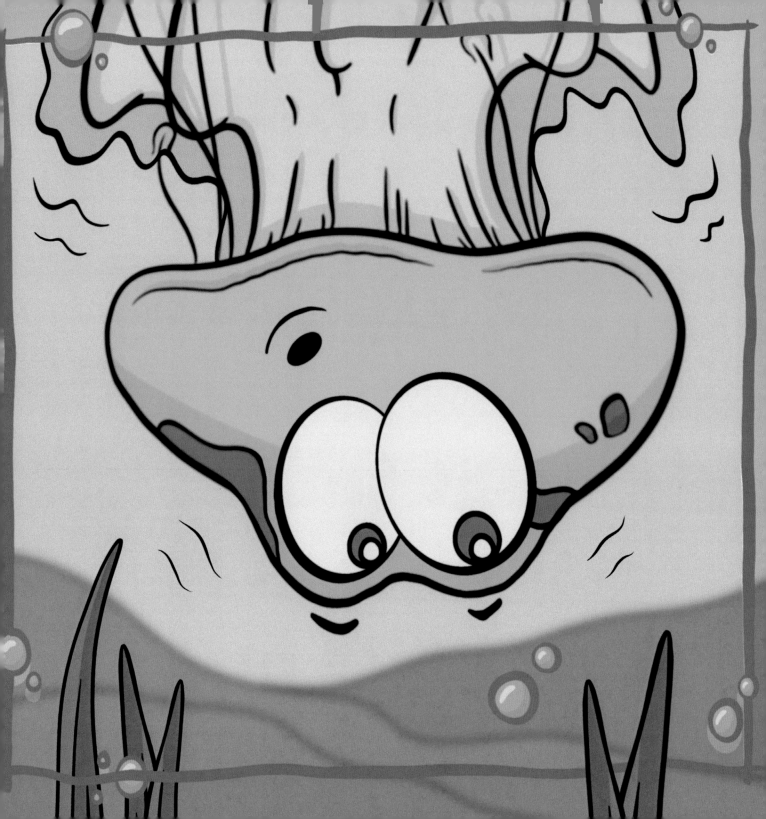

Doc put stickers
on my head
to explain

All that
happens in my
cool little brain

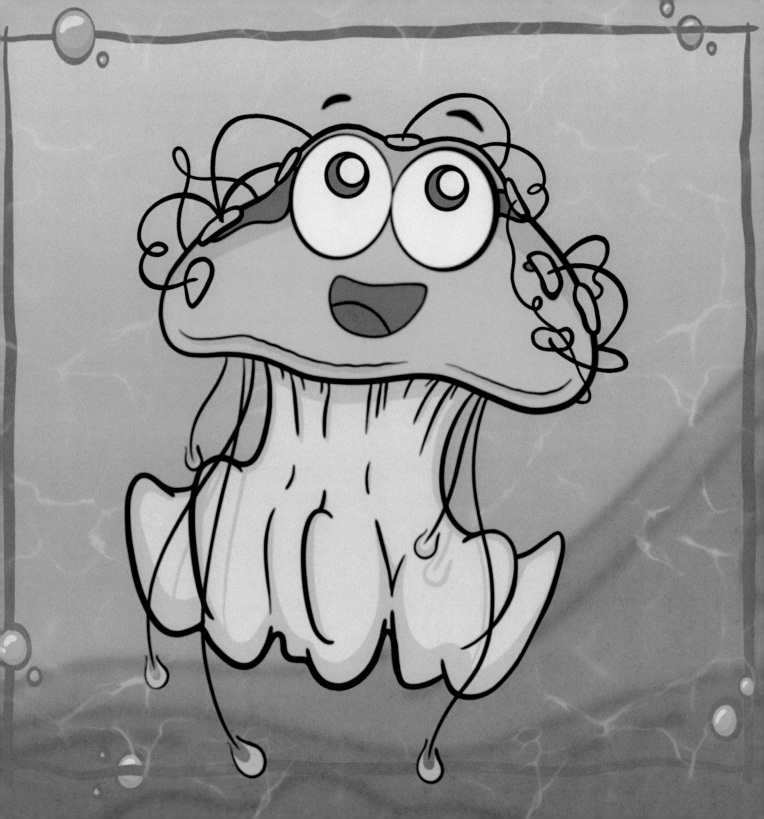

Doc helped me understand my shakes aren't bad,

But I still felt nervous and a little bit sad

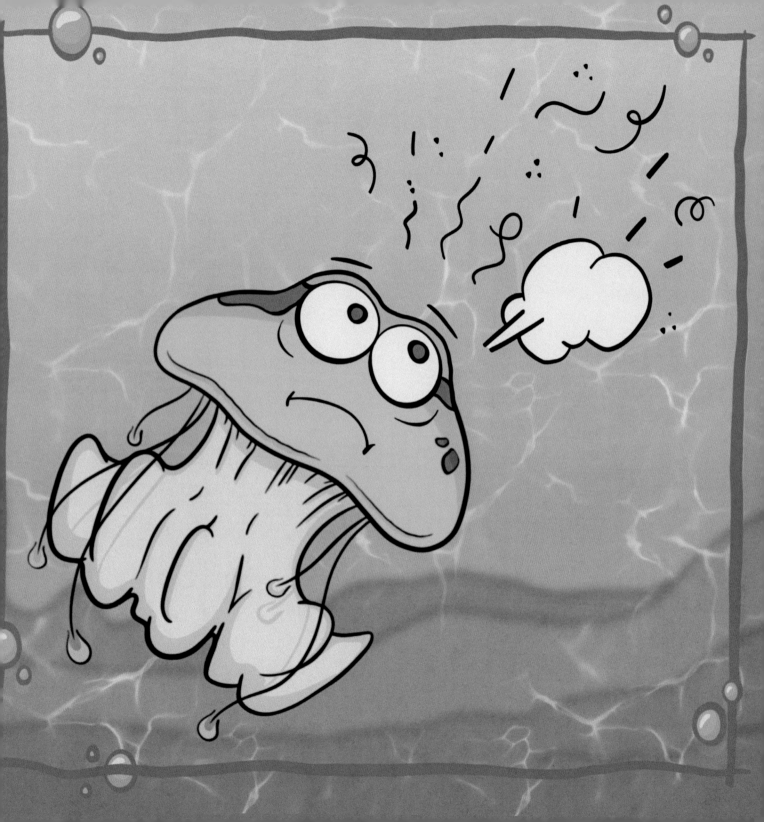

My mom gently told me not to dismay

I didn't do anything wrong - I was just born this way!

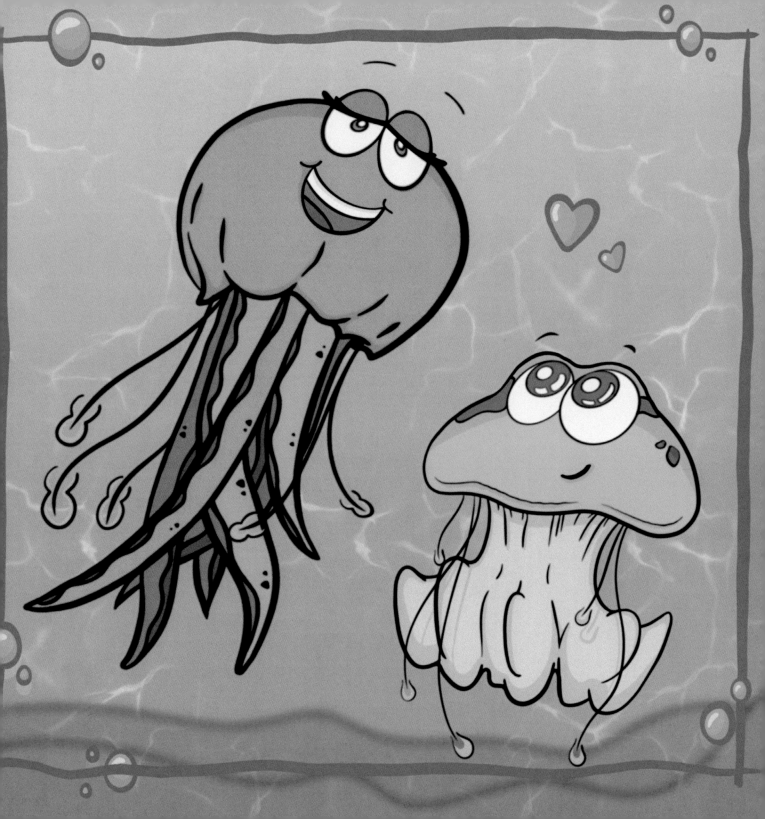

I learned that
my friend Harold
has seizures too

But he shakes a
little differently
than I do

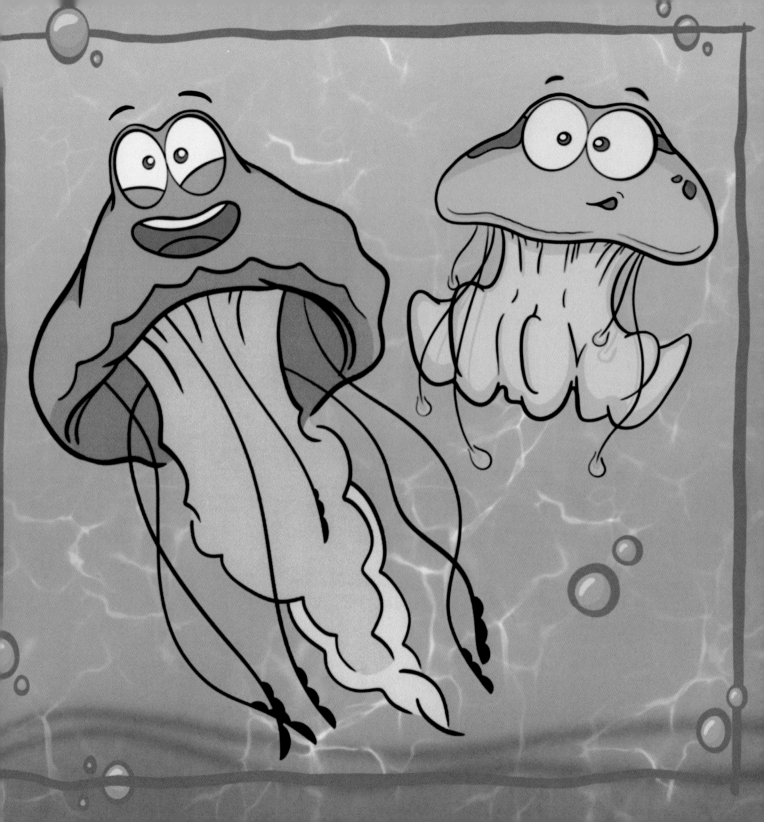

Sometimes seizures don't look like my shakes;

Just like us, they come in all sizes and shapes!

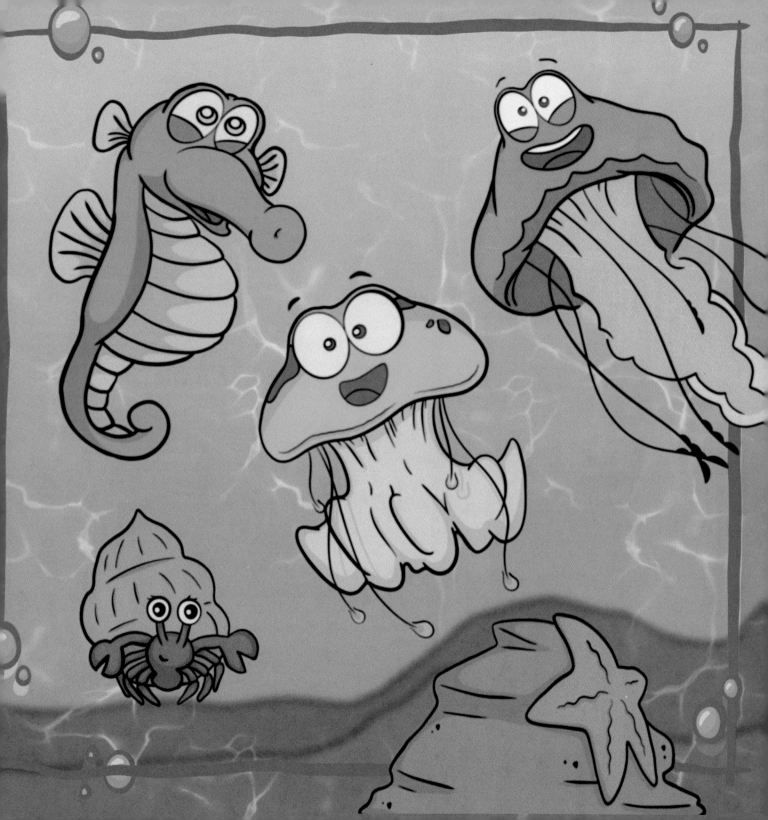

I learned that reducing seizures can help me be a safe guy

Though not all things may help, there are some things we can try

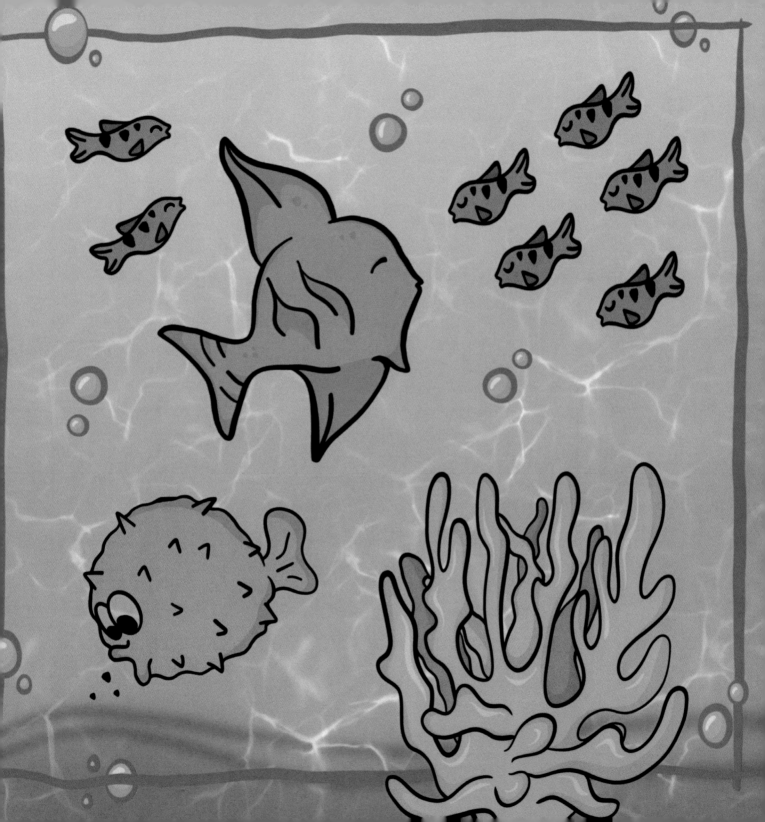

Sometimes Doc Will recommend medicines or certain foods,

sometimes even surgery can help... or a combination of these too!

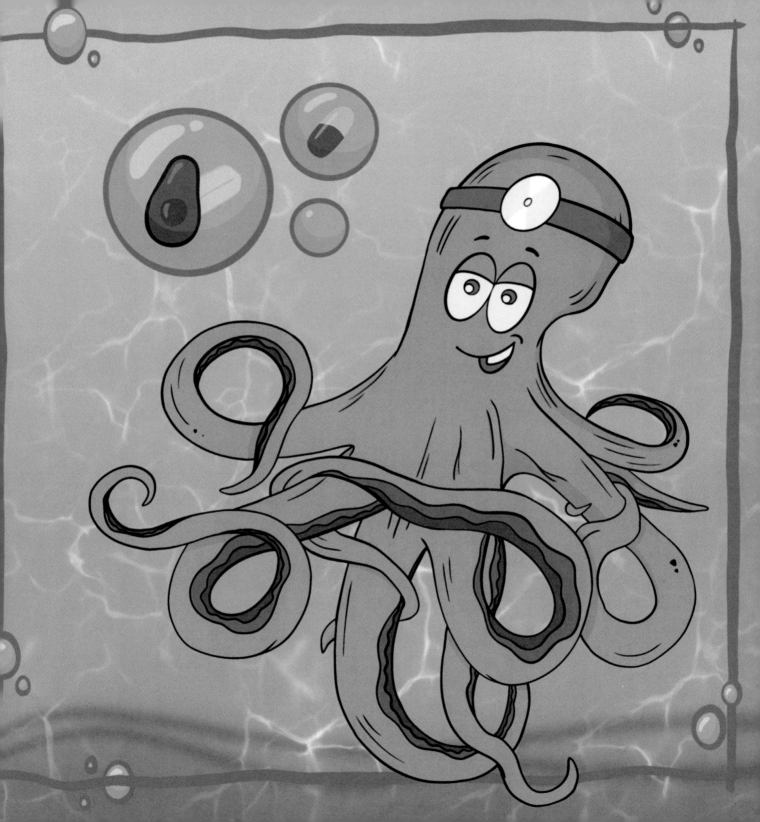

If I do have a seizure in my bed, yard, or pool,

I am kept safe by my family and my friends at school

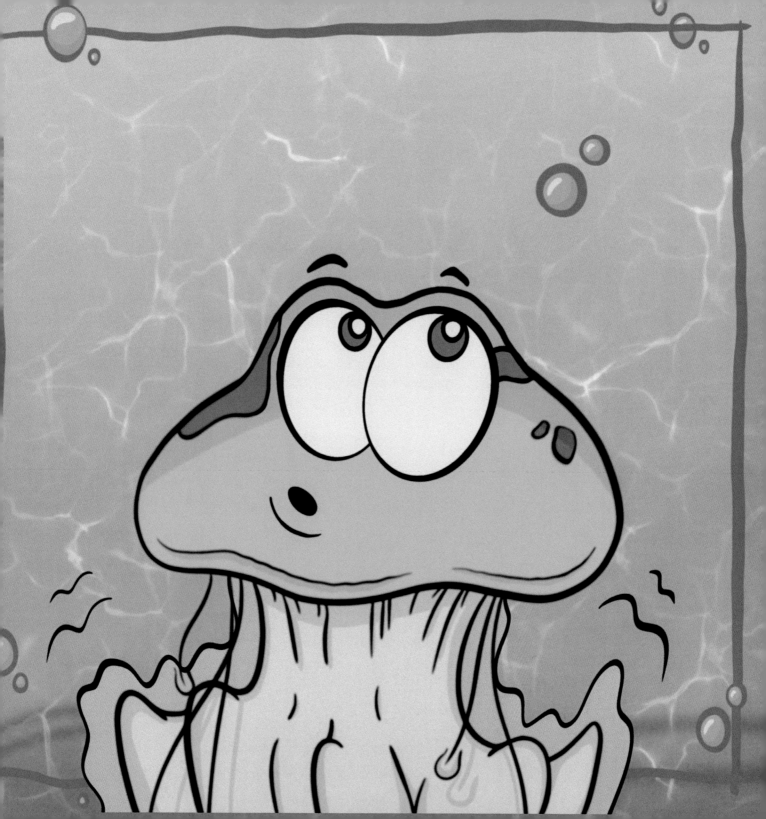

Now I know that
Seizures don't
make me bad or sick,

and I don't have to
fear when they
happen so quick

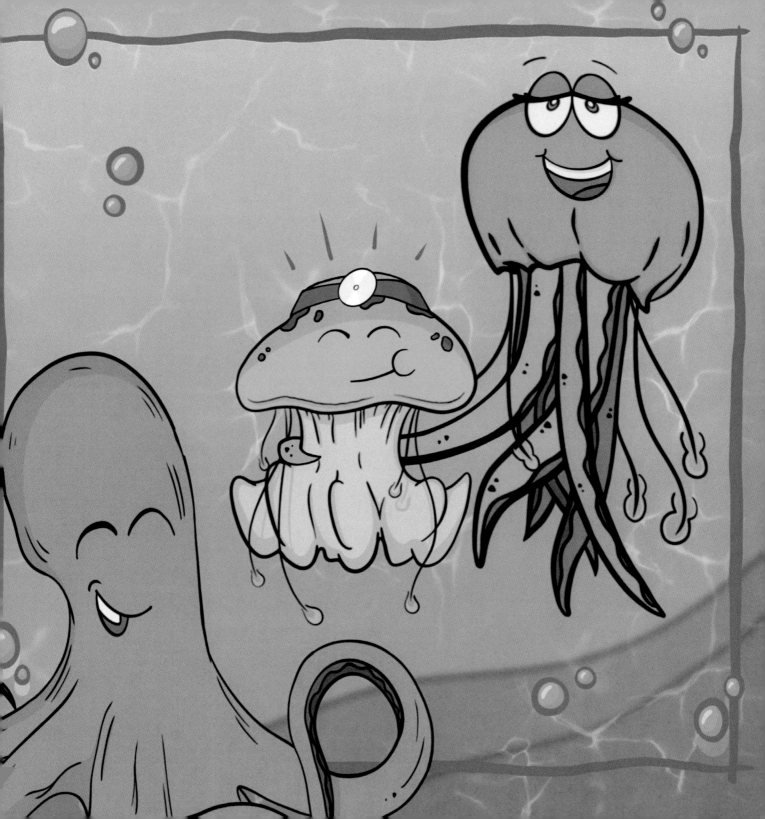

I can play with my friends just like I love to do

I can swim, skip, laugh, and dance, and try new things too!

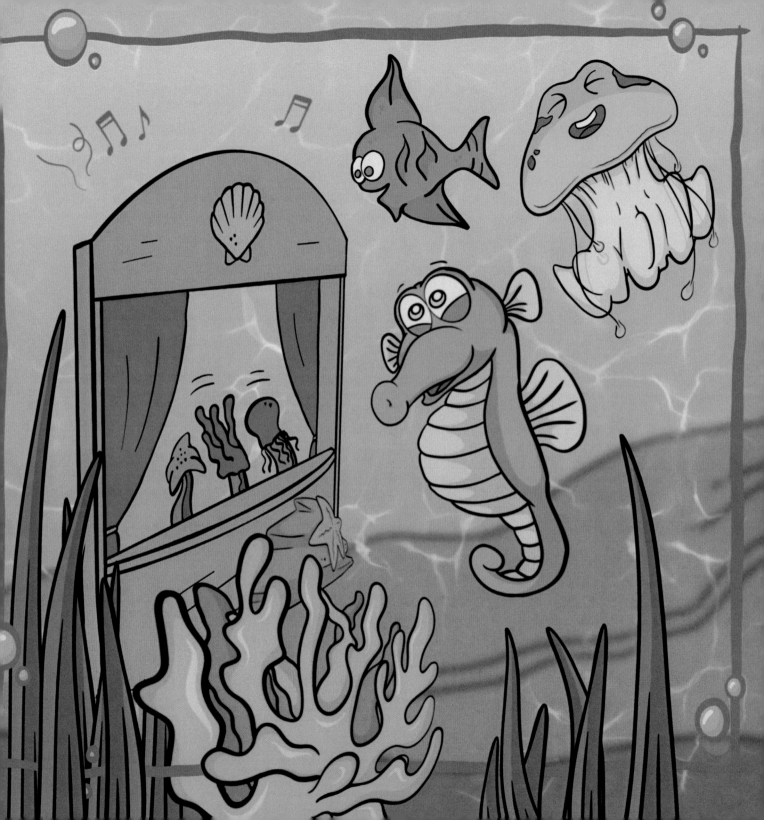

I hope my little story can teach you something new

I get to live a great big life, and I know you can too!

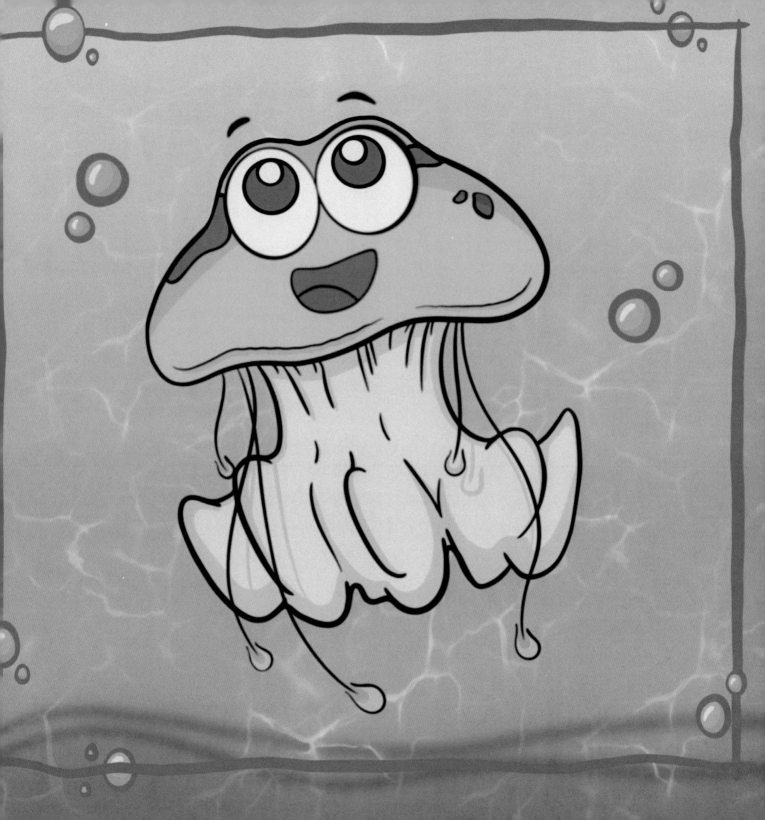

GLOSSARY

Helpful words to learn about seizures

Seizure
A burst of extra electrical activity in the brain
(this can sometimes look like shaking)

Epilepsy
A special condition with multiple recurrent seizures

Electroencephalogram (EEG)
A measurement of electrical activity in
the brain using sensors and a computer

Nervous system
A group of body parts including
the brain, spinal cord, and nerves

Neurologist
A doctor for the brain, spinal cord, and nerves

Seizure precautions
Helpful safety tips to prevent harm when
seizures occur in certain environments

ADDITIONAL RESOURCES

for patients, parents, friends, teachers, & coaches

 scan the codes below for more information!

Epilepsy Foundation	Child Neurology Foundation	Healthy Children
epilepsy.com	childneurology foundation.org	healthy children.org

About the Authors

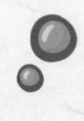

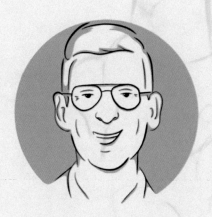

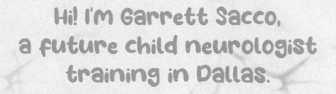

Hi! I'm Garrett Sacco,
a future child neurologist
training in Dallas.

My wife Amy and I created the Brain
Books series to help families faced with
neurological conditions feel informed,
supported, and empowered to live life
fully. I hope this story is accessible and
engaging for you and your loved ones.

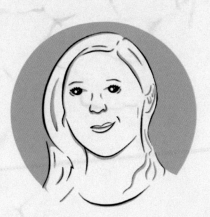

If you enjoyed this book, please pass it
along! If you have ideas for future
stories, let's create one together!

Made in the USA
Middletown, DE
04 May 2023

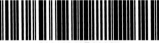

30019340R00027